The Little Book of

Yoga Breathing

The Little Book of

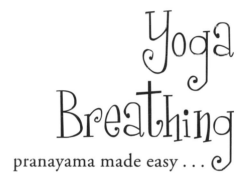

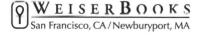

SCOTT SHAW

WEISER BOOKS
San Francisco, CA / Newburyport, MA

First published in 2004 by
Red Wheel/Weiser, LLC
With offices at:
500 Third Street, Suite 230
San Francisco, CA 94107
www.redwheelweiser.com

ISBN-10: 1-57863-301-X

ISBN-13: 978-1-57863-301-2

Library of Congress Cataloging-in-Publication Data
Shaw, Scott.
  The little book of yoga breathing : pranayama made easy / Scott Shaw.
     p. cm.
  ISBN 1-57863-301-X (alk. paper)
  1. Pr—anay—ama--Popular works. 2. Yoga, Ha˘tha. I. Title.
  RA781.7.S4465 2004
  613.7'046--dc22

                              2003017516

Typeset in Adobe Garamond by Kristin Goble

Cover design by Kathllen Wilson Fivel

Printed in the United States
UG

10 9 8 7 6 5 4 3

Table of Contents

Introduction 1

Pranayama 101...7
   Your First Conscious Breath 9
   Breathing Essentials 11

The Energy-Enhancing Breaths 19
   Basic Energy-Enhancing Breath 21
   Kapalabhati: Skull Shining....................25
   Bastrika: Bellows Breathing 29
   Murcha: The Retaining Breath 33
   Kumbhaka: The Pure Breath 37
   Ujjayi: The Hissing Breath 41

The Calming Breaths 45

    Sukha Purvaka: The Easy Breath 47

    Sithali: The Cooling Breath 49

    Sitkari: The Sipping Breath 53

    Brahmari: The Humming Breath 57

    Nadi Sudi: The Nerve-Purifying Breath ..61

Pranayama in Motion 65

    Pranayama While Standing 69

    Leaning Pranayama 73

    Dynamic Tension I: Push the Mountain ..75

    Dynamic Tension II: Lift the Sky 79

    Pranayamic Walking 83

Afterword 89

About the Author..90

Introduction

Modern society moves at such a fast pace that we inevitably find ourselves needing periodic energy revitalization just to keep up with the daily grind. We often try to remedy this with caffeinated drinks or sugar-filled foods. In addition to the obvious health detriments, there are problems with supplementing your energy in this fashion. Though you may be temporarily uplifted, your metabolism will quickly seek to find its own balance, leaving you more drained than ever.

How can you rapidly, healthfully rejuvenate your body and mind in times of need? The natural method, one that instantly provides renewed vigor, is thousands of years old and involves nothing more than taking a few very conscious breaths.

THE ESSENTIAL HUMAN BREATH

The air we breathe is our passport to life. We can live a few days without water, several days without food, but the moment oxygen is taken away from us, our physical bodies immediately begin to pass away. It therefore stands to reason that not only is breathing the most essential element to life, but that breathing correctly will enhance the overall quality of your life.

ENERGIZING BENEFITS OF PRANAYAMA

Modern health science teaches us that through exercise the human body takes in larger amounts of oxygen than is required for simple human existence. This results not only in a stronger cardiovascular system but also a state of enhanced physical and mental health. Look at the athlete who participates in a cardiovascular sport and you'll see someone who possesses a superior sense of physical and mental well-being and an enormous amount of energy. On the other hand, observe sedentary individuals and you'll commonly find people who are listless and lacking motivation.

Though physical exercise is proven to be important to your health, it is not always possible for you to revitalize yourself through exercise—particularly when you find yourself time-crunched and dragging at the end of a workday spent primarily behind a desk. Fortunately, there is another way for you to tap into the energy level experienced by the consummate athlete. That method is known by the ancient Sanskrit word, *pranayama* (pra'-na' ya'ma').

Pranayama is the science of breath control first practiced in India thousands of years ago. The ancient techniques of pranayama teach you how to consciously take control over your breathing and bring more life-giving oxygen into your body. From these simple but precise exercises, you can revitalize your entire being whenever and wherever you feel the need.

The ancient breath control exercises presented here are not abstract metaphysical techniques that will take years of training under the guidance of a spiritual teacher to master. They are simple, proven practices that can be implemented virtually anywhere. Some of them do not even require that you make any physical movements. Therefore, you will be able to perform them in the presence of others without drawing unnecessary attention to yourself.

Using Pranayama to Calm Down

Modern society frequently leaves us needing an energy boost—but it also causes us to become extremely agitated. Many of us find our blood pressure rising and our heart palpitating from the strains of everyday life. The ancient science of pranayama also uses basic methods to rapidly refocus your body and mind and calm down your racing thoughts and emotions. All that is required are a few simple breathing techniques.

Energy-enhancing pranayama exercises are oftentimes the most sought after and practiced. It is important to keep in mind, however, that all pranayamic techniques cause additional amounts of oxygen to be taken into your body in a highly specific manner. As such, though the overall effect of a certain pranayama exercise may cause your body and mind to calm down and become more internally reflective and meditative, this technique will still aid you in becoming a more physically and mentally invigorated individual.

This small book provides you with the necessary information to perform these simple yet very effective breathing techniques. From their practice, you will quickly realize that pranayama has the potential to rapidly change your life for the positive. You will be able to raise your energy level in times of need or calm your body and mind when you need to focus your attention or relax.

Revitalizing your energy and focusing your mind is only a breath away. Breathe on. . . .

Pranayama 101

The Sanskrit term *pranayama* comprises two components: *prana* (life force) and *ayama* (extension). Therefore, the word *pranayama* literally translates as "the extension of life force."

From ancient times forward, we've understood that breathing does even more than supply the body with necessary oxygen for life. When controlled, the inhalation and exhalation of breath purifies and cleanses an individual—and it can calm the agitated mind or energize the overexerted body.

Your First Conscious Breath

The most basic level of pranayama teaches you to simply guide a few breaths deep into your abdomen. This technique is known in Sanskrit as *deergha swasam* (deer-ga'-ha swa'-sa'm)—deep breathing.

There is no time like the present. Right now, wherever you are, breathe deeply. Breathe in through your nose slowly and evenly and guide the air into your abdomen. As you do so, experience your stomach region expanding with the new life force that is inflating your body. After holding this breath for a second or two, release it through your nose at the same pace at which you drew it.

This simple pranayamic exercise will greatly revitalize you when you feel tired, lackadaisical, or stressed—as well as provide an immediate dose of *prana* (pra'-na). Practice this exercise several times every day simply to cleanse your lungs of impurities and realign your inner being with the cosmic energy of prana. Then you can move forward with your life in a much more focused and invigorated manner.

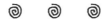

Breathing Essentials

Breathing consciously is your first step to a more refined and energy-filled life. It is essential that you become very aware of your breathing habits to ensure that you are breathing correctly.

Witnessing Your Natural Breath

Begin a conscious analysis of your breathing right now. Close your eyes and take a moment or two to observe your breath as you mentally answer questions on the following page:

1. Are you inhaling through your nose or your mouth?

2. Do your chest and stomach expand or contract when you breathe in?

3. Does your in-breath travel deeply into your abdomen or does it finalize in your chest?

4. What do you feel as life-giving oxygen enters and exits your body?

Now that you have observed your natural breathing patterns, determine if any element needs to be altered and redefined. If you find you are breathing unnaturally, do not become upset with yourself. In each of these cases, unnatural breathing patterns are something that you have simply developed through habit. As such, you can take control and consciously breathe in a manner providing you with enhanced physical and mental energy.

1. Are you inhaling through your nose or your mouth?

If you breathe in through your mouth, you are not allowing your body to naturally filter and purify your intake of air. Airborne pollutants that are not filtered through your nose ultimately end up in your lungs. This is unhealthy.

If you find yourself inhaling through your mouth, correct it by consciously guiding your breath into your body through your nose. With this gentle guidance, your body will eventually adjust to the healthier way of breathing.

2. Do your chest and stomach expand or contract when you breathe in?

If your stomach and chest contract (as opposed to expand) when you inhale, you are breathing unnaturally, hindering the flow of prana into your body. If this is the case, you must take control of your breathing to correct it. Several times a day, take note of your breathing pattern. If you find your chest and stomach are contracting as you inhale, guide your chest and stomach to naturally expand as you breathe in and contract as you exhale.

3. Does your in-breath travel deeply into your abdomen or does it finalize in your chest?

If your in-breaths only travel to your chest, you are not allowing prana to invigorate your body and mind with energy, and you will remain listless and lack energy. Thus, this should be corrected by deliberately reviewing your breathing several times throughout the day—if you invite your breath deep into your abdomen enough times, your body will develop this new, healthier habit.

4. What do you feel as life-giving oxygen enters and exits your body?

By observing what sensations and emotions you experience while life-giving breath is traveling in and out of your body, you raise your consciousness to a new level of understanding. From this position, you interact with the essence of life and how it affects you in all situations. You will become consciously aware of how the quality of the air you breathe affects your body and your overall energy level and recognize when your body is not receiving enough life-giving prana due to polluted or poorly filtered air. You will also realize the point at which your body is not working in natural accord with your respiratory and circulatory systems and either increase your pranayamic or physical exercise to enhance your overall health or break from exercise for a period of time to allow your body to rest.

If you purposely utilize breath awareness throughout the day, not only will you correct any unnatural breathing patterns you've developed, but you will also embrace a more purified state of physical and mental understanding which is essential to a more refined and fulfilled life.

TAKING CONTROL OF YOUR BREATH

Now that you know how to breathe in the most beneficial and natural way, you can advance to the formalized techniques of pranayama. These practices differ vastly from the natural method of breathing described above. In each of the pranayamic breath control techniques that follow, you will be taught to breathe in a highly specific and refined pattern. With each of these techniques you will learn how to consciously take breath into your body while energizing very specific elements of your physical and mental being.

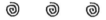

The Energy-Enhancing Breaths

Bringing large amounts of oxygen into your body in a rapid and controlled fashion is not only the most efficient way to instantly increase your energy level, but it is also the healthiest. Whereas all forms of artificial energy stimulation have their side effects, breathing is one hundred percent natural. It is nature's way of giving you the energy boost you need, with no artificial stimuli. All that is required is a few conscious breaths

Basic Energy-Enhancing Breath

Benefits: This breath control exercise will provide you with instant energy revitalization and
enhanced mental focus.

Technique: Begin right where you are. Sit up.
Straighten your spine. Move your neck around a
little bit to relieve any initial tension. Close your
eyes. Observe your natural breathing pattern for
a few moments. Witness each life-giving breath
enter your body though your nose. Mentally
watch it travel deep into your lungs as your
stomach expands. Consciously recognize that
breath is your key to life—it is the universal gift

that allows you to function. Observe this breath permeating your being with the essence of life.

After you have observed a few natural breath cycles, deliberately take in a very deep breath through your mouth. The moment your lungs are full, immediately release it through your mouth. As soon as the breath has been exhaled, take another deep breath through your mouth. Again, once your lungs become full, release it through your mouth.

Practice this for three or four breath cycles and then allow yourself to breathe naturally through your nose for a few moments. As you do, experience how your body instantly became revitalized through the rapid intake of air.

After a few moments of contemplation, take this breath control technique to the next level. Take in a powerful, deep breath through your mouth.

Let this breath expand your chest and stomach. Breathe in as much life-giving air as possible. As soon as your lungs are filled with this breath, close your mouth and hold your breath for approximately two seconds, consciously embracing its power. Now, release this breath through your mouth in one smooth exhalation. Continue to exhale until your lungs are completely empty.

If you are like most people who have not previously practiced formalized breath control, you will notice that a small amount of air remains in your lungs. Through the majority of your life this remaining breath goes unnoticed. Once you begin to consciously practice breath control, however, you become acutely aware of your respiratory system. You must contract your upper abdomen muscles to force the remaining air out of your lungs. With this, you not only expel environmental pollutants that have found their way into your lungs, but you also begin to train your body to utilize the breath in the most beneficial manner—full inhalations and full exhalations.

Once all of the air has been expelled from your lungs, embrace this absence of breath. Experience the lightness of your body when air is completely absent from your lungs. After approximately two seconds of reflection, take in another deep breath and then release it following the same pattern.

Perform this exercise for three or four cycles. Once you have completed your final cycle, open your eyes, observing how the world possesses a new hue due to your body being revitalized by enhanced amounts of oxygen.

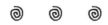

Kapalabhati: Skull Shining

In Sanskrit, *kapalabhati* (ka'-pa'l-a'-bha'-tee) means "skull shining."

Benefits: This exercise is an ancient breath control technique that, when used properly, will not only instantly revitalize your body but will also highly accelerate the degree of your mental awareness.

Technique: While seated, move your upper body and neck around for a few moments to add new circulation to any tense muscles. Then, straighten your spine and close your eyes. Concentrate on your breath and begin to observe the natural energy-giving life force entering and exiting your body through your nose.

When you are centered, take in a very deep breath through your nose. Let this breath fill your lungs. As you do, witness your chest and stomach expand. When your lungs are completely full of oxygen and it is time to exhale, force the air out of your body through your nose with a rapid, powerful push. Immediately inhale again, powerfully, through your nose. As soon as this breath is in, push it out.

Each in-breath and each out-breath in the kapalabhati technique should take approximately one second to execute. You do not hold breath in your lungs at any time during this breath control method. Air is rapidly brought in and then just as rapidly expelled.

At the beginning stage of this breath control technique you should perform three cycles of ten breaths each. At the end of each ten-breath cycle, expel the final breath in a slow and controlled manner. Then, breathe in and out naturally through your nose for approximately three breath cycles. Once the final breath is consciously released, again begin the rapid in and out pattern of breathing.

It is a common side effect in the early stages of this breath control technique for you to become slightly light headed. If this becomes uncomfortable for you, then limit this practice to only one or two cycles. Once your body becomes used to kapalabhati, you can extend this practice for up to ten cycles of thirty breaths each.

Bastrika: Bellows Breathing

The Sanskrit word *bastrika* (ba-streak-a') means "bellows." This word is used in reference to the tool a blacksmith uses to enhance his fire.

Benefits: The benefits of bastrika are rapid energy revitalization and enhanced blood circulation. It also helps your body warm up when you are cold.

Technique: Sit in a comfortable position with your spine straight. Close your eyes for a few moments and watch your natural breathing pattern. When you are suitably focused, close your mouth and rapidly inhale and exhale ten times through your nose. Do not allow these breaths to travel deeply into your body. Instead, allow your breaths to be short and fast. The focus of bastrika is on the exhalation. Like a bellows stoking a fire, allow each in-breath to be rapidly pushed out.

As soon as you have completed your tenth shallow rapid breath, draw a very deep breath through your nose. Allow it to travel into your body. At this point, bend your neck and allow your chin to rest on your chest, thereby holding the prana deeply in your body. Hold this breath and this position for as long as is comfortable. Then, raise your head and fully release the breath. Immediately repeat the entire cycle, starting with the rapid breaths.

Bastrika: Bellows Breathing

Begin the practice of bastrika slowly and gradually, witnessing how your body reacts to this pranayamic technique. In your early stages of practice, bastrika should be performed from one to three full cycles. Become comfortable with it before you extend its practice. If you overdo this exercise you may cause yourself to become light headed. This is, obviously, not to your advantage.

Bastrika is ideally performed for three full cycles. Even by performing this exercise for one cycle, however, you will instantly notice an increase in your energy.

Murcha: The Retaining Breath

The Sanskrit word *murcha*
(mur-cha') means "to retain."

Benefits: The pranayamic technique of murcha is designed to enhance your mental energy and to provide you with a subtle sensation of euphoria.

Technique: Sit down in a comfortable position, close your eyes, and take in a few very conscious, deep breaths through your nose. Do not hold these breaths. Simply allow them to enter your body and be released in a natural pattern. This will immediately enhance your level of energy and cleanse your lungs.

When you feel you are mentally ready, draw another deep breath through your nose and guide it deeply into your body. This time, hold it. As you did in bastrika, bend your neck, bringing your chin down to your chest if possible.

Hold this breath and bodily position for as long as is comfortable. Then, raise your head and release the breath through your nose. As soon as this breath is completely expelled, repeat the cycle, starting with a deep breath through your nose.

As in all pranayamic techniques, it is essential to never strain your body. Murcha should be performed from one to five breath cycles. Do not hold your breath longer than is comfortable. As you progress, the amount of time you can comfortably hold your breath will naturally be extended.

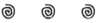

Kumbhaka: The Pure Breath

In Sanskrit, *kumbhaka* (kum-bha'-ka') refers to "pure breath."

Benefits: Kumbhaka is designed to subtly raise both your physical and mental energy. In addition, kumbhaka provides the practitioner with a heightened sense of mental and spiritual awareness.

Technique: Begin in a seated posture. Close your eyes, straighten your spine, and focus your attention upon your natural breathing pattern for a few moments. As you do, concentrate your mind upon the energy that each in-breath naturally provides.

When you feel ready, close off your right nostril with your right thumb. Quickly and deeply draw your next breath through your left nostril. Rapidly draw the breath deeply into your body with a mental count of "one, two, three, four, five, six."

The moment your inhalation is complete, immediately release this breath via your left nostril (the same nostril from which it was inhaled). As you expel this breath, perform the same mental count of "one, two, three, four, five, six." Be sure to consciously push any remaining air out of your lungs.

When this breath has been completely released, experience the emptiness of no breath for a mental count of "one, two, three, four, five, six, seven, eight, nine, ten, eleven, twelve."

When your count is complete, change sides—close off your left nostril with your left thumb and begin the process on the opposite side.

It is important to not strain or fatigue your body. When you begin to practice this pranayamic technique, it should be performed for three cycles—even less if you find that three repetitions are too many. As you progress with this technique, increase repetitions to as many as twenty.

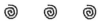

Ujjayi: The Hissing Breath

In Sanskrit, *ujjayi* (u-jai-yee) means "hissing," the sound you make when performing this technique.

Benefits: Ujjayi is designed to subtly enhance your energy and leave you feeling not only more invigorated but also more mentally focused. From a metaphysical perspective, ujjayi cures the body of respiratory ailments such as asthma and bronchitis.

Technique: Sit down, straighten your spine, close your eyes, and witness your natural breathing for a few moments. When you feel ready, very consciously take a deep breath in through both of your nostrils. Allow this breath to travel into your body. As you inhale, mentally lock this breath in the region between your central chest and your throat.

Retain this breath for as long as is comfortable. When it is time to exhale, do so by closing off your right nostril with your right thumb and exhaling through your left nostril.

Once the breath is completely released, immediately draw another breath through both of your nostrils. Allow it to congregate in the same region as your previous breath—between your central chest and throat.

Again, hold this breath for as long as is comfortable and then release it. As you do so, close off your left nostril with your left thumb and exhale via your right nostril.

Ujjayi should be performed from ten to twenty repetitions, depending on your time constraints, at the early stages of its practice. When you are comfortable with this pranayamic exercise, increase to fifty or more repetitions. This is an ideal exercise to perform in the morning on a day when you know your energy levels will be put to the test.

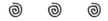

The Calming Breaths

When you begin the practice of pranayama, remember that enhancing the overall energy of your body does not only occur when you are feeling invigorated. At times, calming down is the best way to focus and regenerate your energy. Perform the following pranayamic exercises when you need to become more insightful and subtly rejuvenate your energy.

Sukha Purvaka: The Easy Breath

Sukha purvaka (sue-ka' purr-va'-ka')
means "the easy breath" in Sanskrit.

Benefits: Sukha purvaka is designed to quickly
calm your mind and lower your cardiovascular
rate in times of stress. It is also an excellent technique to practice prior to meditation, as it
invokes a clear and positive state of mind.

Technique: While sitting comfortably with your
hands in your lap, close your eyes, straighten
your spine, and watch your breath naturally

come in and then leave your body. Embrace the life-giving force of each breath.

When you feel ready, close off your right nostril with your right thumb. Inhale slowly and naturally through your left nostril. When your in-breath is complete, allow this breath to leave your body naturally, also through your left nostril. Perform this exercise for twelve breaths.

When you have completed your final exhalation, place your right hand back down in your lap, raise your left hand, and close off your left nostril for the same twelve natural breaths. When you have completed this repetition, place both hands in your lap and relax for a few moments. You will rise in a very calm state of mind, and your mental clarity will be acutely focused.

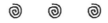

Sithali: The Cooling Breath

In Sanskrit, *sithali* (ʒit ha' lee) is
the "cooling breath."

Benefits: Use this pranayama exercise to physically cool down your body when it is exposed to high temperatures. It is also used to remove the desire for food, water, and sleep when they can not be had.

Technique: Sit down, close your eyes, and observe the natural incoming and outgoing process of your breathing for a few moments. Once you have achieved a relative state of calm, curl your tongue in a circular pattern and extend it outside of your mouth. As you breathe, bring the air in through the central passageway. Do not force your in-breath but consciously take it in, while mentally witnessing prana feeding your entire being. As the final part of your inhalation is reaching completion, bring your tongue inside of your mouth and close your lips. Hold the breath for as long as is comfortable. Then, release the breath through your nose.

Experience the light feeling of emptiness gained from the absence of air in your lungs for a moment or two until you feel that it is time to breathe. Once again, extend your curled tongue and slowly breathe in.

Perform this pranayama technique for up to fifteen breath cycles. It can settle your mind and fulfill the immediate needs of your body so you will not be distracted by cold, thirst, hunger, or fatigue when accomplishing a physical or mental activity.

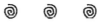

Sitkari: The Sipping Breath

In Sanskrit, *sitkari* (sit-kar' ee) means "sipping," the sound you make performing this technique.

Benefits: Sitkari is a breath control technique designed to quickly calm your body and mind while invigorating your mental capacity. Sitkari is a cleansing breath, as is the previously detailed sithali—it keeps you from experiencing cold, hunger, and thirst, while providing you with additional energy

The Calming Breaths

Technique: This pranayamic exercise is performed by initially sitting down and consciously settling into your seat. Straighten your spine, close your eyes, and observe your natural breathing patterns for a few moments. When you feel ready, place your tongue firmly against the upper palate of your mouth. With your next inhalation, slowly breathe in through your mouth. This will cause the incoming air to make a sipping sound. Once your in-breath is complete, relax your tongue, close your mouth, and hold the breath in your lungs for as long as is comfortable. Then, release it via your nose. With your next in-breath place your tongue against the top of your mouth again and breathe in through your mouth, again making the sipping sound.

Sitkari: The Sipping Breath

Practice this technique between five to ten repetitions to calm your body and mind and center your being upon any task that needs to be accomplished.

Brahmari: The Humming Breath

In Sanskrit, *brahmari* (bra'-ma'r-ree)
means "the humming breath." This
refers to the sound you make as this
pranayamic technique is performed.

Benefits: Brahmari is a calming breath control
technique that quickly steadies a troubled mind.
Brahmari also activates the higher realms of the
personal self. It is a great exercise to perform
prior to meditation as it enables the mind to
become very clear and focused.

The Calming Breaths

Technique: Sit down, close your eyes, and take in a few focused breaths, slightly deeper than you would normally breathe in. Allow your mind to focus and become calm. When you feel ready, begin by breathing in through your nose. As you do so, contract your glottis (the opening between your vocal chords). This creates a snoring sound as the breath enters. Once this in-breath has filled your lungs, hold it for as long as is comfortable and then release it through your nose. Continue your exhalation until the breath has completely exited your body. You can aid this process by pushing any remaining air out of your body with your stomach muscles, if you find it necessary. Once this has been accomplished, experience the natural emptiness for a few moments and then breathe in again following the previously detailed pattern.

Brahmari: The Humming Breath

This pranayamic technique should be practiced for approximately ten repetitions as a means to center and focus your mind.

Nadi Sudi: The Nerve-Purifying Breath

In Sanskrit, *nadi sudi* (na'-dee suit-ee) means "the nerve-purifying breath."

Benefits: Nadi sudi is the essential body and mind calming exercise. There is no pranayamic technique more well suited to quickly calm the racing mind and slow the accelerated heart rate.

Technique: Sit down and allow yourself to relax and reflect for a few moments. When you feel ready, close your eyes and take a deep breath.

Hold this in-breath for as long as is comfortable and then consciously release it.

Place your right hand up to your nose and close your right nostril with your thumb. Inhale slowly yet deeply through your left nostril. Observe your breath slowly enter and flow into your body in a stream of calming energy. Once your in-breath is complete, allow it to remain in your lungs for five seconds. Slowly count "one, two, three, four, five." Now, open your right nostril by removing your thumb from it. At the same time, close your left nostril by placing your forefinger against it. Allow the breath to, slowly and naturally, flow out from your body through your right nostril. Once your breath has completely exited, feel the serene emptiness. Count, "one, two, three, four, five."

When it is time to breathe in, inhale through your right nostril. Hold it, as previously described, for the count of five. When the time of breath release has come, close off your right nostril with your thumb, open your left nostril, and allow the breath to slowly exit via your left nostril.

Repeat this process approximately twenty times. Nadi sudi quickly brings about a lightness of body and a calm and focused mind. It is an ideal technique to perform before entering into meditation or going to sleep.

Pranayama in Motion

Traditional pranayama was once thought to solely be a method for zealots to cleanse the various aspects of their physical and spiritual being while nourishing themselves with prana in order to gain a deeper state of meditation and ultimately experience enlightenment. As such, the majority of the traditional pranayama exercises were designed to be practiced from a stationary or seated posture.

As the science of pranayama has evolved over the centuries, the traditional exercises have laid the foundations for new, more active techniques. Modern practitioners may now incorporate ancient breath control techniques into virtually any physical movement in order to enhance their physical and mental well-being.

In the modern world, where so many people are locked to their desks all day long, many forget just how beneficial a little movement can be. Certainly, science has taught us that formalized physical activity is essential to the reduction of stress and the enhancement of physical and mental health. But, in many cases, it is difficult for modern individuals to break away from their daily grind to exercise.

Hatha yoga has long been known to rejuvenate the body and mind. But while hatha yoga requires you to accomplish formal postures, more common physical movements can raise your energy level—when performed with breath control. Mental focus is essential to take pranayama to the level where formalized breath control techniques are integrated with movement. You must remain extremely conscious of not only your breath but also your body at all times whenever you integrate pranayama with movement.

Pranayama While Standing

Benefits: Standing pranayama is a method of rapidly infusing your being with additional amounts of prana, proving you with additional energy to take on any task at hand. It is also a great source of body/mind coordination.

Technique: Stand up and loosen your neck by slowly moving it around in a circular pattern. Increase the blood flow into your hands and arms by moving them around. Put your hands on your hips and rotate your upper body from the base of your spine. Continue these movements for a few moments and consciously take notice of the increased blood circulation within your body.

When you feel ready, leave your hands on your hips, close your eyes, and take in a couple of deep breaths through your nose. Experience these breaths traveling deep into your body. Release these breaths in a natural pattern, through your nose, when you feel it is time to do so.

Now, deliberately straighten your spine. With your eyes remaining closed and your hands still on your hips, take in a deep breath through your nose. As this breath comes in, allow your body to lean backward at the base of your spine. Let your head also lean backward until the rear of your skull rests on your upper back. (Be careful not to lean back too far, as you do not want to lose your balance.)

When your intake of air has reached its climax, relax and hold this position for a few moments. Feel the revitalizing energy of the oxygen held in your body.

As you release this breath, slowly move back up to a natural standing position. When you are again erect, breathe for a few natural breath cycles. Watch these breaths entering your body, as you embrace their life-giving power. When you feel ready, lean back with your next in-breath.

As every pranayama technique is about body/mind consciousness, so too is this one. Therefore, lean back in association with the intake of your breath. Make leaning back a process of awareness. Your lean should begin at the outset of your in-breath and culminate when your in-breath is complete.

Perform this exercise up to five times to refocus your body and mind, causing the natural effects of movement and added oxygen intake to regenerate your physical and mental being.

Leaning Pranayama

Benefits: As with standing pranayama, leaning pranayama is both a tool for body/mind coordination and energy revitalization.

Technique: Stand up and move your body around to loosen any muscle tension and to get your blood flowing. Take in a couple of deep breaths through your nose, causing new prana to enter your being.

Close your eyes and separate your feet farther apart than normal, about shoulder width. Allow your arms to hang naturally loose and at your

Pranayama in Motion

side. Observe your natural breathing patterns for a few breath cycles.

When you are ready, take in a deep breath through your nose. Hold this in-breath only for a second. Immediately, lean to your right side. Allow your right arm to naturally move away from your body. As you lean, expel this breath in three distinct exhalations through your nose. As soon as the breath is fully released, bring your body up to an erect position and immediately take in a new deep breath through your nose. Again, hold this breath only for a second, and release it in three distinctive spurts as you lean to your left side.

Perform this invigorating pranayama technique up to ten times to vitalize your body and mind with new pranic energy and provide you with the ability to focus your mind upon mentally trying tasks.

Dynamic Tension I: Push the Mountain

Dynamic tension exercises are a method of very consciously tightening the muscles of a specific region of your body. Advanced athletes who wish to develop a very defined muscle group commonly use this method of exercise. More than just a method for muscle growth, however, dynamic tension causes additional blood flow to circulate throughout your body. Therefore, these exercises, used with pranayamic breath control, can instantly invigorate your body and mind.

Benefits: This exercise is an ideal tool to not only tone your body but also to refresh your mind and energy in times of need.

Technique: Begin in a standing position with your hands loosely at your sides. Close your eyes and observe your natural breathing pattern for a few moments. Start when your mind is focused and prepared to be receptive to incoming life-force energy.

Take in a very deep breath through your nose. When your in-breath is complete, hold it in your abdomen as you count to ten. Then release the breath through your nose.

Upon its complete exhalation, breathe in slowly and deeply through your nose and take a step forward with your left leg. As you continue to inhale, bend your elbows and raise your hands until your open palms are facing away from you at chest level. Hold this breath for a count of ten.

Now, as you exhale through your mouth, tighten the muscles of your shoulders, back, arms, and hands. Powerfully push forward with your open palms, visualizing a mountain in front of you moving with the power of your push.

Once this breath is completely exhaled, hold your position for a ten count and experience the absence of breath. Leave your arms extended in front of you and witness how your blood circulation has substantially increased in your arms, shoulders, upper back, and legs, causing a new invigoration of energy to pulsate throughout your body.

When it is time to breathe again, inhale as you step forward, swinging your right leg in front of your left and bringing your open palms back to their beginning position at your chest. Hold this breath for a count of ten.

When it is time to exhale, again push the mountain as you extend your palms from your chest. Once you've exhaled, hold your position for a count of ten and experience the absence of breath.

Perform this dynamic tension pranayama exercise up to ten times. It will give you new life and empower your hands, arms, and upper body.

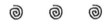

Dynamic Tension II: Lift the Sky

Benefits: As with push the mountain, this exercise is an ideal tool to tone your body and revitalize your energy.

Technique: Begin in a standing position with your legs at shoulder width and your hands naturally to your sides. Close your eyes. Loosen any tension in your body by moving your head, upper body, and arms around slightly.

Once you are ready, settle into your positioning and observe your natural breathing pattern for a few moments. Now take in a very deep breath through your nose. Hold it as you count to ten, then release the breath through your nose.

Inhale again through your nose while bringing your hands up alongside your body. When they reach shoulder level, face your palms to the sky. Hold this breath for a count of ten as you experience its life-giving power.

When it is time, exhale though your mouth. As you exhale, begin to push upward with a powerful yet controlled upper body movement. Mentally see yourself pushing the sky upward. Your arms should reach their most outstretched point upon the completion of your exhalation. Experience the powerful emptiness of this lack of air in your body as you count to ten.

Now, as you slowly inhale, bring your arms down to your side and then back up to shoulder level upon the completion of your inhalation. Hold this breath for a count of ten and again push the sky as you exhale.

Perform the lift the sky exercise for five breath cycles. Not only will your mind become acutely focused but your body will also be empowered with newly revitalized energy.

Pranayamic Walking

Benefits: By its very nature, walking is a prana-inducing activity. When you walk, you safely increase your cardiovascular rate and your body begins to naturally take in more life-giving oxygen. You quickly become more energized and take this energy with you throughout the rest of your day.

Though many people walk for fitness, pranayamic walking is not power walking to primarily burn calories and enhance endurance. You are walking to link your body and mind to the more meditative elements of life. This also provides your body with necessary fitness, which naturally enhances your energy.

Some teachers suggest performing certain styles of pranayama exercises, such as kapalabhati, while walking. Though possible, associating this style of pranayama with walking has the potential to set your body out of balance and cause you to hyperventilate. As such, this is not an ideal form of practice.

As you begin your first pranayamic walk, think about the fact that although you have walked an untold number of miles in your life, how often have you been aware of your breathing while walking? This is what sets the pranayamic walk apart from average walking.

Technique: To begin, simply set a destination and start walking. As you start this journey, take note of your breathing. Witness how you breathe more rapidly as your body warms up and your blood flow increases.

Many people naturally begin to breathe through their mouths when they walk. It is easier to breathe through your mouth during cardio-aerobic activities because oxygen may be more readily taken in. To bring the practice of prana-yama walking, however, you must control the way in which you breathe.

First, deliberately breathe in and out solely through your nose. By consciously breathing in this fashion, you use your body's natural filtra-tion system. Of course, if at any point this becomes difficult, breathe through your mouth and simply slow down your walk.

MOVEMENT MEDITATION

By consciously observing your breath as you walk and deliberately inhaling and exhaling through your nose, you elevate walking to the level of a movement meditation. It is no longer simply a voluntary physical activity.

By walking in this fashion, you naturally become very aware of how prana enters and exits your body. You notice how the incoming air invigorates and empowers you. It becomes very evident when air is absent from your body. Not only are you exercising your body, but you are also reaching a new level of mental refinement in your quest to remain energy-filled in times of need. From this practice in consciousness you understand how to most effectively take prana-filled oxygen into your body when it is needed.

THE MIND AT PLAY

Once you become aware of your interaction with prana-filled oxygen, it is natural to toy and experiment with its various effects. You may find yourself holding your breath a bit longer than is necessary, or consciously taking deeper breaths than are required. This is not necessarily bad. In fact, the great thing about breathing, especially when you are in the midst of a physical activity, is that if you are not breathing correctly, your body will quickly take control over the process and force you into a more natural pattern. Through this experimentation, you will ultimately come to a new and more refined understanding of life-giving prana entering your body through breath, allowing you to harness this essential energy in times of need.

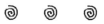

Afterword

For centuries, pranayama techniques have been taught, practiced, and expanded upon, leaving little doubt of their substantive value. Those of us who inhabit this modern world are no longer required to focus our pranayamic practice solely upon sought-after enlightenment. Instead, we can take these ancient exercises, place them in a modern perspective, and use them to address the needs specific to our time in history. Pranayama may become the tool that aids each of us in making our ultimate contribution to the evolution of humanity.

All you have to do is breathe. . .

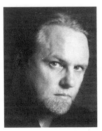

Scott Shaw is an accomplished writer, teacher, martial artist, and practicing Buddhist. He has been teaching yoga for over twenty-five years and is the author of many books, including *Yoga: The Inner Journey*, *About Peace*, *Zen O'clock*, *Tao of Self-Defense*, and *Nirvana in a Nutshell*.